THE IMMUNITY SOLUTIONS FOR YOU!

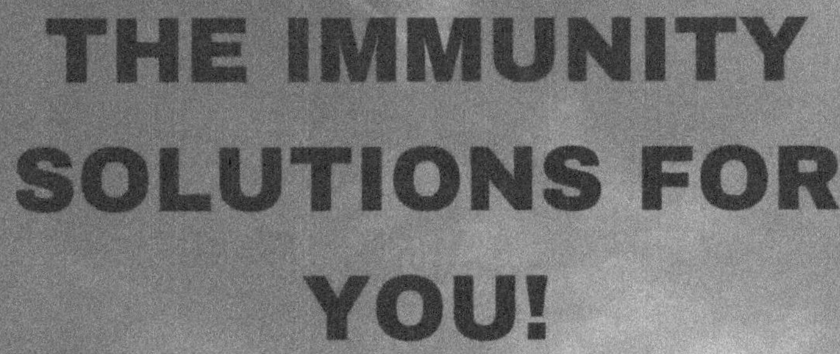

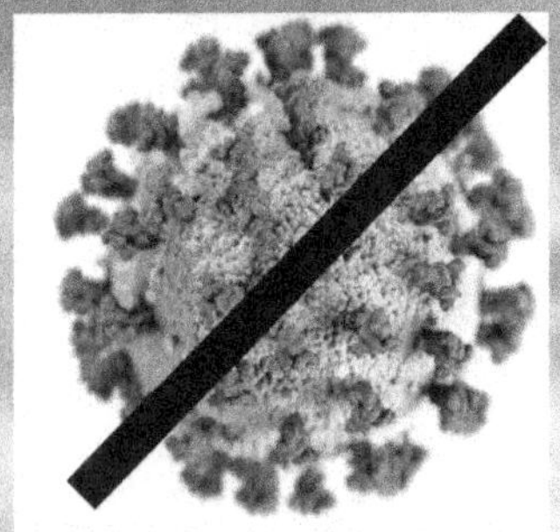

Step-by-step guide to understanding how the immune system functions and strengthening it

SURESHA PARASHIVAMURTHY

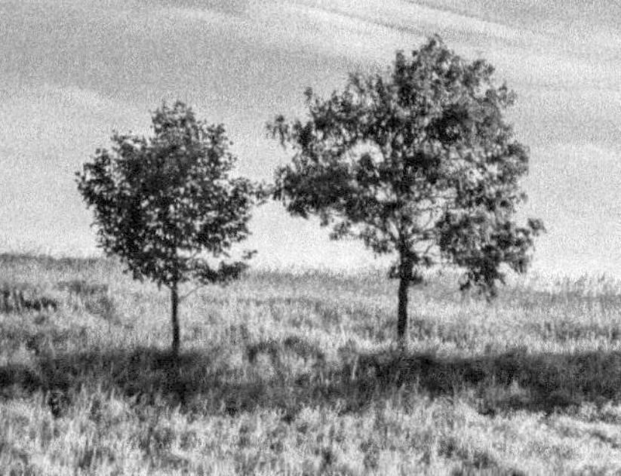

THE IMMUNITY SOLUTIONS FOR YOU!

Step-by-step guide

Suresha Parashivamurthy

SP

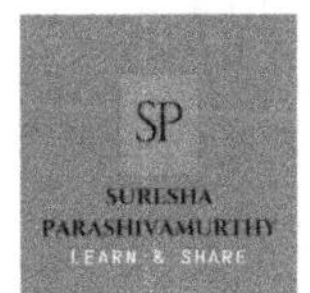

Copyright © 2021 Suresha PARASHIVAMURTHY

All rights reserved

The characters and events portrayed in this book are fictitious. Any similarity to real persons, living or dead, is coincidental and not intended by the author.

No part of this book may be reproduced, or stored in a retrieval system, or transmitted in any form or by any means, electronic, mechanical, photocopying, recording, or otherwise, without express written permission of the publisher.

LEGAL DISCLAIMER: The author wholly owns this book's copyrights. The author has made every reasonable effort in the creation of this book to be as accurate and complete as possible; however, the author/publisher/reseller assumes no responsibility for any omissions, errors or contrary interpretation of the subject matter herein and does not warrant or represent at any time that the contents within are accurate or complete and does not replace any professional medical treatement.Any website, product, and company names mentioned in this report are their respective owners' trademarks or copyright properties. The author/publisher/reseller is not associated or affiliated with them in any way. COMPENSATION DISCLOSURE: Unless otherwise noted, the links in this book are shared only for knowledge purposes. The author/publisher/reseller will not receive a fee or benefits. The author/publisher/reseller, on the other hand, disclaims all liability that might arise as a result of your interaction with such websites/products. Before purchasing the goods mentioned above or services, you should conduct due diligence. Any disagreements or terms not addressed in this agreement are at the publisher's absolute discretion.

Cover design by: Suresha PARASHIVAMURTHY

FOREWORD

Your immune system is a fantastic machine. It's responsible for keeping your body safe from outside invaders like viruses, bacteria, fungi, and toxins.

Your immune system is divided into two parts: the part you were born with (innate or non-specific system) and the function you create due to environmental exposure (adaptive acquired or specific system).

Your immune system comprises various organs, cells, and proteins – skin cells, blood, bone marrow, tissues, and organs like the thymus and lymph glands. A robust immune system is your best defense against illness and infection. Without it, you would have no way of fighting off harmful substances or changes within the body.

This book is an attempt to share different methods we can improve immunity naturally.

CONTENTS

INTRODUCTION

Your immune system is a marvel. It protects the body from foreign invaders such as viruses, bacteria, fungi, and toxins.

Your immune system is divided into two parts: the part you were born with (innate or non-specific system) and the function you create due to your exposure to the environment (adaptive acquired or specific system).

The immune system comprises proteins, several organs, and cells like the thymus and lymph glands.

A balanced immune system is the most robust defense against illness and infection. With good immunity, you all be able to fight dangerous chemicals or changes in your body.

Your best protection against disease and infection is a healthy immune system. You wouldn't be able to fend off toxic substances or changes in your body if you didn't have them.

Three primary functions of the immune system:

1. To eliminate pathogens (disease-causing "germs") such as viruses, bacteria, fungi, and parasites from your body.
2. To combat disease-causing changes in the body, such as cancer cells.
3. To recognize and neutralize toxic substances in the environ-

ment.

Antigens – substances that your body doesn't accept as belonging there – cause your immune system. Bacteria, viruses, and fungi all have proteins on their surfaces.

When your immune system cells come into contact with these antigens, they cause a cascade of events in your body.

Once you come into contact with a germ, it will identify it if re-encountered in the past and release antigens. During this scenario, vaccines are effective in protecting you from such diseases.

There are five indicators that your immune system might use a boost.

When your immune system is out of whack, not everyone notices — mainly if you're used to feeling lousy! Here are a few indicators that your immune system could use some help:

1. You get sick sometimes, and your colds last a long time.

2. After sufficient rest, you're still tired.

3. Eczema and other skin conditions that cause dryness

4. Consistent digestive problems

5. You're allergic to a variety of stuff.

What factors contribute to a compromised immune system?

There is no simple explanation for why one person's immune system is superior to another's.

Though genetics play a role, evidence suggests that the environment (i.e., lifestyle factors) has a more significant influence on the immune system than genes.

The following are examples of "risk factors" that can contribute to a weakened immune system:

A sedentary way of life

Sleep deprivation

High levels of anxiety

A high-carb, high-sugar diet

In this book, we'll look at the best all-natural and healthy immune boosters that anyone can use to improve their immune system, increase their resistance to disease and infection, and help them heal faster if they do get sick.

Let's get started!

1.EXCERCISE

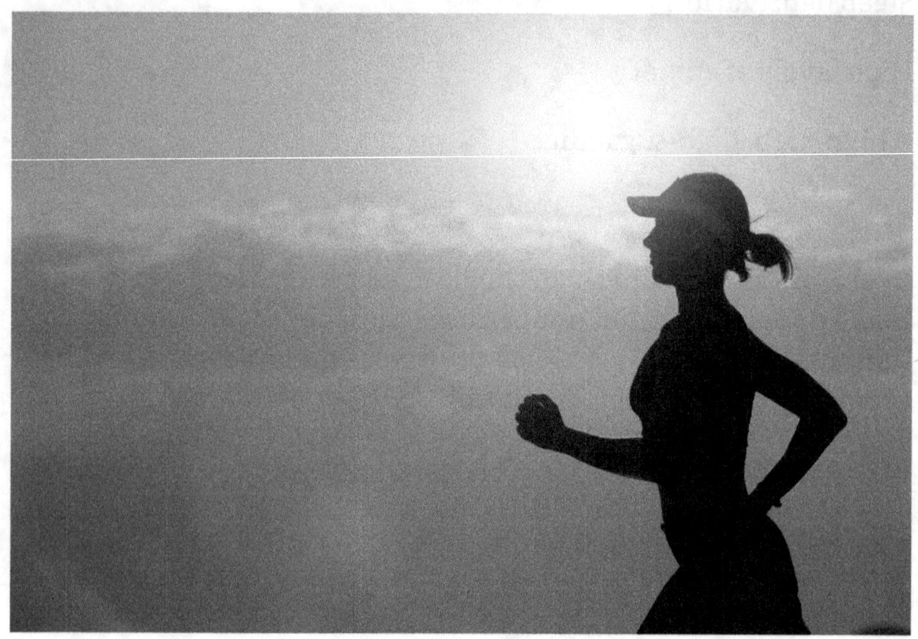

On the other hand, moderate exercise was shown to improve the immune response compared to prolonged vigorous exercise. Even one session of moderate exercise, according to studies, will enhance vaccine efficacy in people with weakened immune systems.

"Exercising is an excellent way to strengthen your immune system," says the author.

Exercise speeds up the circulation of the antibodies and white blood cells, allowing them to detect germs more efficiently. "Being involved in this way often decreases stress hormones, lowering the risk of getting sick."

According to a new survey, people who exercised at least five days a week had half the risk of getting a cold as someone who did not.

Daily moderate exercise can also help to minimize inflammation, linked to improved immune function. Training will also aid in the normal regeneration of the immune cells.

30 to 60 minutes of fast walking, jogging, biking, steady bicycling, and light hiking three to five days a week are examples of moderate exercise.

It's worth noting that the majority of these are associated with the outdoors. There's a good reason to exercise outdoors, particularly if you're deciding between outdoor and indoor exercises.

T-cells, which are particular parts of your immune system that help you combat infection, can be stimulated by sunlight. Being outdoors also exposes you to phytoncides and other plant products that can help your immune system. It also increases the body's Vitamin D levels, which aids your immune system even more.

To maintain your fitness, you can do strength training exercises twice a week.

Three main types of excercise which will help to improve immunity are as follows:

Strength training - Strength training is a form of exercise that consists of movements designed to increase the body's strength and endurance. Here's a short rundown of how muscles grow in size and strength.

You're applying a new stressor to your working muscles in this case, your stomach, arms, and shoulders — if you've never done a pushup before and only do one rep. As a result, the muscle tissues suffer micro-tears, which the body's will heals to adapt, and muscles grow bigger and stronger as a result. Only the most straightforward variations of exercises can elicit a reaction if you're new to strength training, and as you get stronger, you can raise the weight, reps, and sets to keep improving.

<u>Hiking and Walking -</u>

Aren't you sure ready for strength training? Take a stroll. We don't need research to warn us that being indoors and glued to our phones is bad for us, but it does. Despite the social distancing rules in effect, you can go outside, which is something you can do because it helps you feel better.

A study linked 90-minute bouts of outdoor walking to lower activity in the part of the brain linked to depression. Trail hiking's more rugged terrain raises your workout intensity while still allowing you to see more of nature.

<u>High-Intensity Interval Training or HIIT</u> - involves doing an exercise as hard as you can for a specified period (usually 20 to 60 seconds) and then relaxing for the same amount of time. You'll raise the heart rate much higher and much quicker than you can with slow and steady exercise. It's pretty strenuous, but a HIIT session usually only lasts around 15-20 minutes.

If it's been a while since you've exercised regularly, start with light strength training and walking and work your way up to HIIT. It's very intense. However, it's the strength of your workout that causes an "afterburn" effect, in which your body continues to burn calories for hours after you've finished.

So, you should exercise regularly and get enough sunlight to boost your immune system and increase your overall health.

2. PLANT BASED FOODS

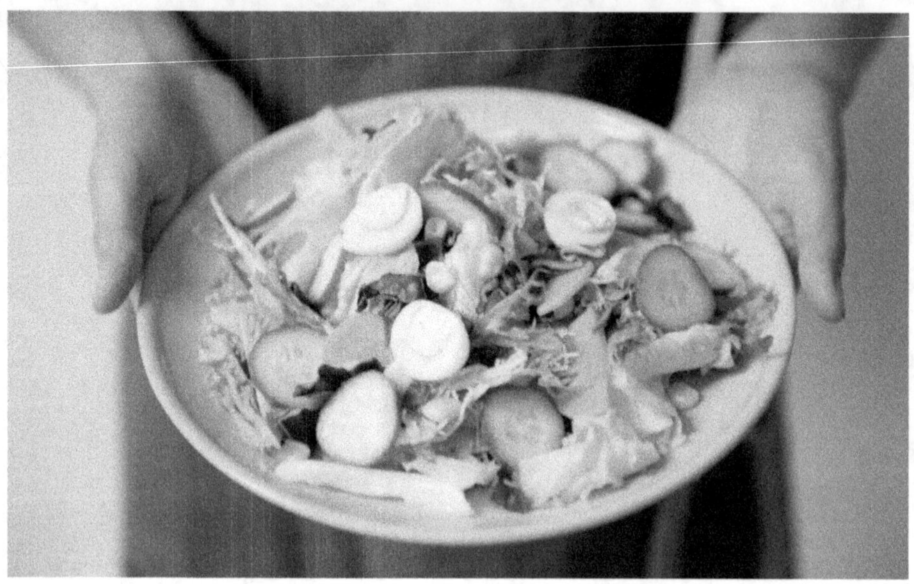

Inflammation in the body is a significant cause of today's refined diet. Our forefathers consumed more raw fruits and vegetables, and doctors have shown that this is a better diet for your immune system (as well as other systems in your body).

Antioxidants and nutrients contained in whole plant foods help to improve the immune system. Consume a diverse range of foods, with fruit and vegetables of every rainbow color as a goal.

Fresh fruits and vegetables are much healthier for you than refined foods and supplements, but eating a rich diet is not only artistically pleasing.

Protein is for immune system function. A low-protein diet can reduce your body's ability to fight infection because amino acids help create and maintain immune cells.

Vitamin C, Vitamin B6, and Vitamin E are the three most important vitamins for your immune system.

One of the essential vitamins that your immune system needs are Vitamin C. Since your body does not store Vitamin C, you must consume enough of it through your diet.

Your kidneys empty everything you don't need out of your body.

The good news is that you can get enough Vitamin C without wasting money on supplements by eating various foods. Citrus fruits (and their juice), strawberries, bell peppers, broccoli, kale, and spinach are good sources of Vitamin C.

Another immune-boosting vitamin is B6, also known as pyridoxine. Since it's a water-soluble vitamin that your body doesn't make, you'll need to eat the right foods to get enough to keep your immune system healthy.

Chicken or turkey and cold-water fish such as salmon or tuna are all excellent sources of B6. Green vegetables and chickpeas can also include Vitamin B6 (the main ingredient in hummus). So, even though you're a vegan, you can get enough B6 to keep your immune system in good shape.

Vitamin E is an effective antioxidant and fat-soluble vitamin. Nuts, seeds, and spinach all contain it. It would help if you were more cautious with Vitamin E because it is included in your fat and can build up to harmful levels.

Vitamin E supplements to be prescribed by your doctor.

If you're older or feeling especially tired, you should get your Vitamin D levels checked by your doctor. The majority of people get enough Vitamin D by simply going outside, where sunlight increases the body's production of the vitamin.

If your doctor recommends it, taking 400 IU every day is shown to boost disease-fighting cells such as T-cells. Vitamin D found in fatty fish such as tuna, mackerel, and salmon, as well as beef liver, cheese, and egg yolks.

Zinc, folate, iron, and selenium are additional nutrients that your immune system needs, according to the Academy of Nutrition and Dietetics.

While getting these nutrients from food is preferable to taking supplements, they are necessary to help your immune system. Increasing whole plant foods will significantly boost your immune system.

Ginger -

Did you drink ginger ale whenever you were sick at home when you were a child? The aim was fine, but the execution could use some support. Instead of soda, which contains many inflammatory refined sugars, go straight to the source: ginger! Because of its high antioxidant content, ginger is beneficial to the immune system.

Favorite ginger-based immune-boosting recipes:

Soup with Spicy Carrots

Pad Thai with Almond Ginger

Tea with ginger and turmeric

Beets -

Beets help in the improvement of gut health. A healthy stomach leads to a healthy immune system in many cases. Beets make your tummy happy because they contain a lot of fiber, which is good for digestion. Fiber keeps you regular, feeds good bacteria in your gut, and protects you from digestive illnesses like inflammatory bowel disease and diverticulitis. It's a resounding victory!

Favorite beet-based immune-boosting recipes:

Sandwich with Peanut Butter and Beets

Roasted Beets with No Oil

Garlic -

Garlic used to treat colds for decades, so it isn't just an urban legend. Here's where science comes into play! Garlic contains allicin compounds, which improve immunity and reduce inflammation.

Even better, you don't have to eat raw garlic cloves to benefit from their medicinal properties.

Our favorite garlic-based immune-boosting recipes include:

Garlic Ginger Broccoli

Lemon Garlic Oil-Free Dressing

Oil-Free Garlic Hummus

Turmeric -

Turmeric isn't just good for reducing inflammation; it can also boost your immune system's efficiency. Curcumin, the yellowing agent in turmeric, also stimulates T cells and other pathogen-fighting cells in the body, making it easier to avoid illness.

Our favorite turmeric-based immune-boosting recipes include:

Turmeric Latte

Healing Winter Soup

Lemon Lentil Soup

Mushrooms -

When it comes to improving the immune system, mushrooms are unrivaled. Vitamin D is abundant in them (which activates the immune system response and helps T cells do their warding off infection). They also contain beta-glucans, which stimulate killer cell activity, which may aid in the prevention of illness.

Our favorite mushroom-based immune-boosting recipes include:

Plant-Based Pesto Stuffed Mushrooms

Vegan Mushroom Tetrazzini

Tamari Mushroom Stuffed Sweet Potato

Oranges, Kiwis and Strawberries -

While we all know that Vitamin C is beneficial to our immune systems (hello, antioxidants!), don't reach for the orange juice just yet. Refined sugars found in orange juice, which may induce inflammation in the body. Instead, seek out whole food sources. Oranges, strawberries, and kiwis are among our favorite vitamin C-rich fruits.

Our favorite Vitamin based immune-boosting recipes include:

Chocolate Covered Strawberries

Carrot Orange Soup

No-Bake Kiwi Vegan Cheesecake

Oatmeals -

You can't go wrong with oatmeal when it comes to your diet. Oats are beneficial for various reasons, including weight loss, cardiovascular health, cancer prevention, and digestion. They're high in fiber (which is good for your gut!). Oats also contain zinc, an essential nutrient for your immune system since it aids the proper functioning of T cells and natural killer cells.

Our favorite oatmeal-based immune-boosting recipes include:

4-Ingredient Vegan No-Bake Oatmeal Cookies

Chewy Oatmeal Banana Pancakes [Gluten-Free]

Oatmeal Muffins

3. SLEEP

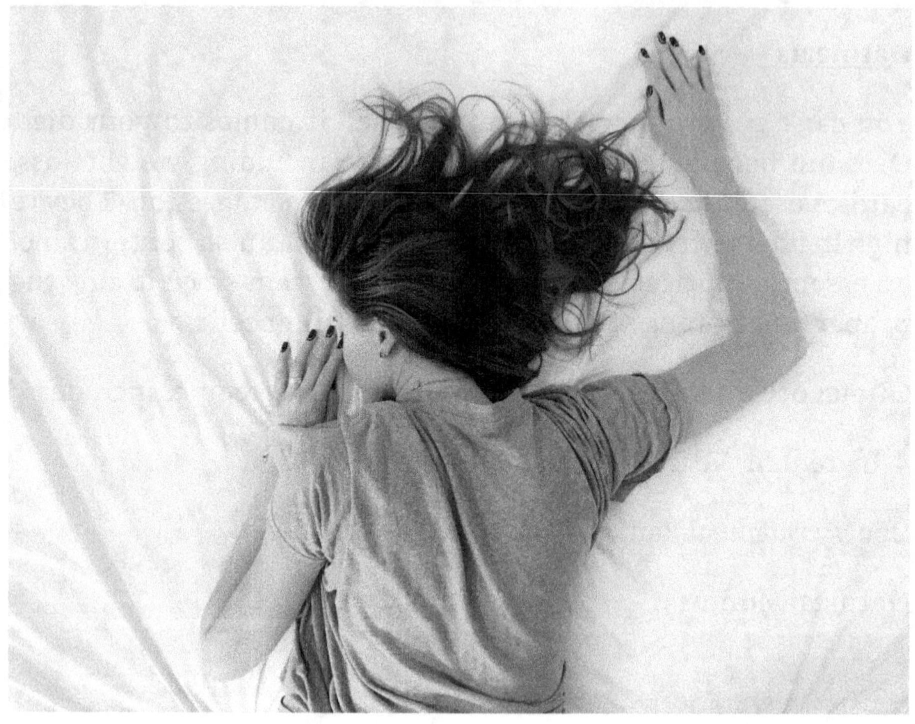

Sleep deprivation will lower your immune response, making you more susceptible to infection.

A survey found that those who slept less than six hours per night were more likely to catch a common cold.

Your body produces stress hormones like cortisol to keep you awake and alert, suppressing your immune system, When you don't get sufficient sleep.

You can also take longer to heal if you haven't had enough sleep. That's because if you don't get enough rest, your body won't produce enough antibodies to combat the disease.

Your body also produces specific proteins (cytokines) that help your immune system, but only when you're sleeping.

In sleep, the body heals and regenerates. To work correctly, most adults should get seven or more hours of sleep every night..

Adults need a minimum of eight hours of sleep every night, while younger children and infants require up to 14 hours.

According to a report, people who got eight hours of sleep had more T-cells than those who slept less. A study discovered that people who get seven hours of sleep are four times less likely to catch a cold.

Most modern people don't get enough sleep, which is unfortunate because it's a simple solution to a common issue.

Limiting screen time a minimum of two to three hours before bedtime is one of the best ways to get a decent night's sleep. Shut down the TV, computer screen, and cellphone because blue light is shown to interrupt the body's normal sleep cycle (circadian rhythm).

We should also be kept caffeine to a minimum. If you're having trouble sleeping, consider cutting out caffeine afternoon. Even if you think your body is used to it, a little caffeine can go a long way.

You can try sleeping in a completely dark, cooler-than-the-rest-of-your-house bed as your body cools down when it's time to sleep.

Often, avoid reading or having stimulating talks right before bedtime. They raise your adrenaline levels, making it more difficult to calm down.

Except on your days off, go to bed simultaneously every night and stick to a sleep routine before going to bed.

Speak to your doctor if you're still having trouble sleeping.

A good night's sleep is essential for a healthy immune system and many other body systems. You won't be able to function at your best if you don't get enough sleep.

Steps to Strengthen Immunity from sleep with the following habits:

<u>Consistency in sleep:</u>

One of the most critical aspects of having a good night's sleep is consistency. Our bodies become used to a routine, just like any other habit.

Waking up and going to bed at the exact times every day helps your body establish a sleep pattern. Maintaining a regular sleep schedule can also be achieved by avoiding naps during the day.

<u>Hormones and Sleep Consistency</u>:

Hormones are released and recovered in a predictable pattern in your body and brain. The routine release of a variety of hormones affects overall health. These hormones are released in different ways and at other times, depending on how much sleep you get.

Our modern lifestyles contribute significantly to our sleep deprivation, but regular, high-quality sleep is an essential component of living a long, safe, and happy life.

Light:

Our circadian rhythms, or internal body clocks, have been programmed to respond to light, synchronized Human sleep-wake cycles with the sun's natural day-to-night period until the advent of electricity-powered artificial lighting. Our brain releases melatonin when the sun sets, and it becomes night, which makes us feel tired and helps us sleep. Our eyes and skin release chemicals that allow us to stay awake as the sun rises the following day. As a result, even a tiny amount of artificial light during the night will disrupt sleep.

Blue light:

Blue light induces alertness, keeps our brain awake, and blocks the development of melatonin. The screens (phones, computers, and televisions) we like to look at right up until we try to fall asleep emit blue light.

Our sleep cycle is also affected by LED lights and fluorescent bulbs. At least one hour before bedtime, restrict your exposure to these forms of light. Blue light mitigating filters or glasses can be beneficial, but it is best to switch off all devices before bed.

Screen Filters for Devices that Reduce Blue Light:

Blue light reduction filters are integrated into several smartphones, televisions, and computer monitors. You can also program your phone to go into this mode at a specific time.

Eyeglasses that reduce blue light:

Consider having blue-light filtering eyeglasses if you don't have, or don't want to spend the money on, newer electronics with blue light filters. If you wear glasses, you can consider adding a blue-light filtering coating to your next pair.

Aromatherapy will help you relax:

Aromatherapy will help to sleep better and relax. Lavender is a familiar fragrance that improves sleep quality and reduces anxiety.

The scent of cedarwood can help you sleep longer and avoid waking up too early. Like rosemary or sandalwood, some smells can be stimulating, so keep them out of aromatherapy blends. Pillow sprays, pressure point roll-on applicators, and space diffusers all contain these essential oils.

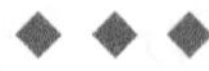

4. HYDRATION

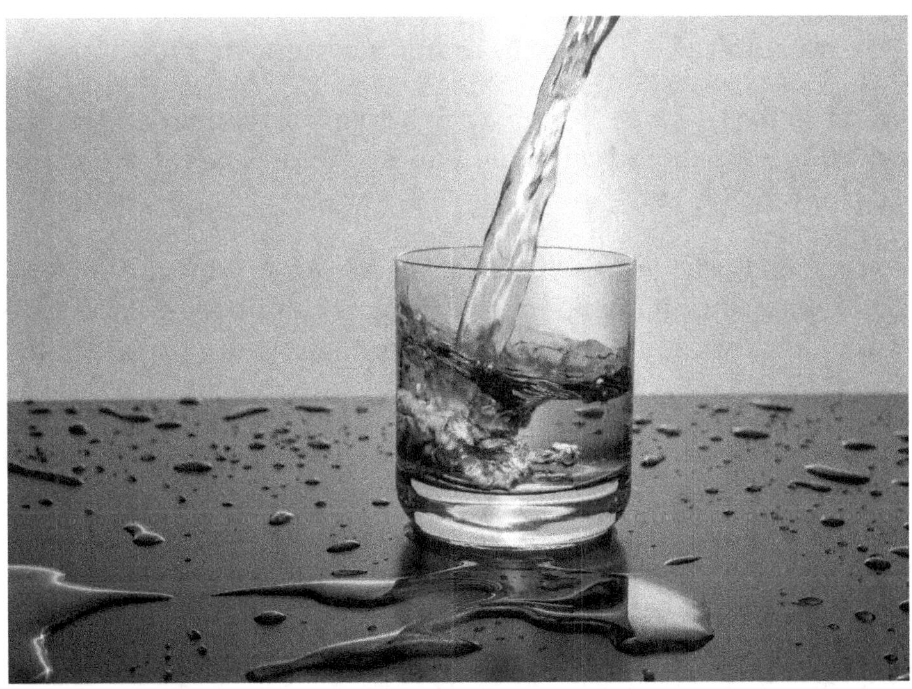

When the body did not get enough water, it becomes dehydrated. Physical performance, mood, concentration, digestion, and heart and kidney function may all be affected. These can also reduce the disease resistance.

The first sign that you're not getting enough water is a familiar sensation called thirst. There's a chance you'll get a headache as well.

You should drink enough water to produce pale yellow urine. Water is the safest option since it contains no additional calories.

Try to limit the intake of sweetened beverages such as fruit juice, sweet tea, and sodas. Although this will help you stay hydrated, the added sugar will suppress your immune system and counteract the benefits of consuming enough water.

Staying hydrated will help the immune system function better.

Water helps to make lymph, which transports immune system cells like white blood cells. Cucumbers, melon, and celery are hydrating foods to eat.

As a general rule, you can drink if you're thirsty and continue to do so until your body no longer requires liquid. If you exercise, work outdoors, or live in a hot environment, you can need more fluid.

As you get older, your body cannot communicate your need for water, so you're less likely to drink enough. Even if you don't feel thirsty, if you're over 55, you can make sure you drink plenty.

While hydration has no direct effect on your immune system, it is beneficial to your overall health and, as a result, to your immune system.

<u>Significant benefits of drinking water helps to strengthen immunity:</u>

Water Helps Your Body Remove Waste

Water Aids In Digestion And Prevents Maladies

Water Prevents Dehydration

Water Helps Your Brain Function Optimally

Water Keeps Your Cardiovascular System Healthy

Water Protects Your Joints, Spinal Cord And Tissues

Water Helps You Produce Saliva

Water Helps Regulate Your Body Temperature

There are different ways to boost our water intake and hydration to enhance our immunity:

Alkaline water:

The term "alkaline" refers to a pH range. This scale, which ranges from 0 to 14, determines how acidic or basic a substance is. The pH of alkaline water is between 8 and 10.

The acidity of alkaline water differs from regular water, which means it contains more hydroxide than hydrogen ions.

Minerals such as magnesium, potassium, and calcium are alkaline. It is well known for its ability to neutralize harmful substances in the body.

Furthermore, alkaline water is quickly absorbed by your body, enabling it to make the best use of the water you drink.

Aside from that, the following are some of the recognized health benefits of alkaline water:

Strengthens the immune system

Enhances the effectiveness of your circulatory system

Strengthens bones and improves blood flow

Aids digestion and absorption.

Removes toxins

Antioxidant properties are present

Assists in the treatment of gastroesophageal reflux disease

Warm Water:

Although the water of any temperature is beneficial to overall health, warm water has several additional advantages.

It aids in the faster digestion of food, resulting in better digestion.

Warm water causes sweating, which contributes to the release of toxins, which detoxifies the body.

Warm water improves blood circulation by dilating blood vessels. This relieves tension and relaxes the muscles.

Warm water aids weight loss by increasing metabolism, absorbing nutrients, and flushing waste.

It aids in the removal of nasal and throat obstruction by allowing mucous to pass more quickly.

Lemon Water :

Lemons are loaded with a variety of nutrients like magnesium, calcium, iron, fiber, potassium, B-complex vitamins, and vitamin C. They contain more potassium than grapes or apples.

It can help your body in the following ways:

Wards off diseases and infection.

Improves your immune system.

Helps with wound healing.

Lemon water helps the body to absorb iron from foods.

Adds a dash of flavor to your water so that you can switch out your sugary dose with lemon water. Lemon helps restrict calorie intake and potentially promotes weight loss.

The citric acid in lemon juice can also kill the bacteria that causes bad breath.

The high vitamin C content helps prevent free radicals from causing cell damage, leading to cancer.

Lemons assist in the formation of collagen, which helps maintain healthy .

It can help relieve or prevent nausea.

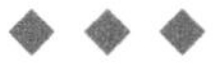

5. HEALTHY FATS

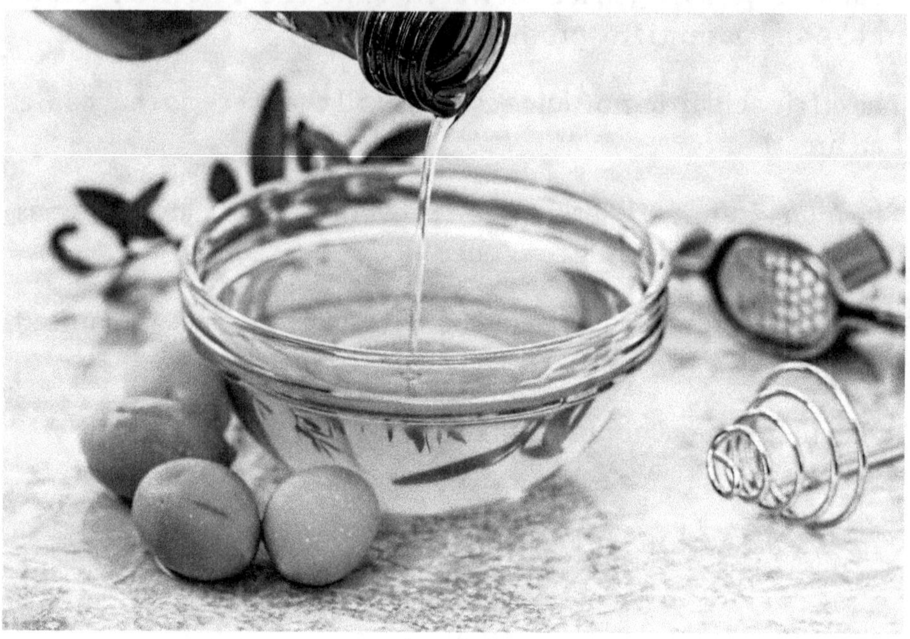

Our stomach contains 80% of your immune system. so when it's safe, we're able to combat infections faster and better. When it isn't, our immune system is weakened, making us more vulnerable to infection.Anti-inflammatory fats, such as olive oil, nuts, and fatty fish like salmon, are considered healthy fats.

By reducing inflammation, can help your body's immune response. Chronic inflammation, such as that caused by a high-fat, heavily refined diet, suppresses the immune system's responses.

In research, olive oil has been linked to a lower risk of type 2 diabetes and heart disease.

It has anti-inflammatory properties and can help the body fight harmful viruses and bacteria.

Omega-3 fatty acids, found in cold-water fish like salmon and chia seeds, have also been shown to minimise inflammation and improve immunity.

In general, the study suggests that people follow a Mediterranean diet. This entails a diet high in fruits, vegetables, whole grains, and good fats. She says, "This eating pattern is rich in nutrients like Vitamin C, zinc, and other antioxidants help minimize inflammation and combat infection."

Adults aged 65 to 70 who ate a Mediterranean-style diet had minor increases in disease-fighting cells (T-cells).

Healthy fats can help stimulate your immune system and boost your body's response to disease or infection.

Plant-based foods with an optimum omega-3/omega-6 ratio and high levels of linoleic and alpha-linolenic acid include:

Hemp seeds contain 30% fat, with 80 percent of omega-3 and omega-6 fatty acids. Protein, magnesium, and potassium are all abundant in them.

Walnuts are high in omega-6 fatty acids and contain a healthy amount of omega-3 fatty acids. Walnuts are often rich in antioxidants, which help the immune system significantly.

One tablespoon of Chia Seeds contains 2,282 mg of omega-3 and 752 mg of omega-6 fatty acids!

Although dark leafy greens are low in fat, they have an excellent omega-3 ratio.

Two tablespoons of flax seeds contain 3,600 mg of omega-3 fatty acids! Beans, especially mung beans, have a very favorable omega-3 to omega-6 ratio, with omega-3s weighing 15 times as much as omega-6s.

In just one cup of cabbage, particularly cauliflower, you'll get 208 mg of omega-3 and 62 mg of omega-6. Winter squashes, especially butternut and acorn squashes and pumpkins, are high in omega-3 fatty acids.

Acai Berries have a higher concentration of polyunsaturated fatty acids than other fish. This antioxidant-rich superfood boosts the immune system's efficiency. A single ounce of wakame seaweed contains 52 mg of omega-3 fatty acids and is an excellent source of iodine.

6. PROBIOTICS

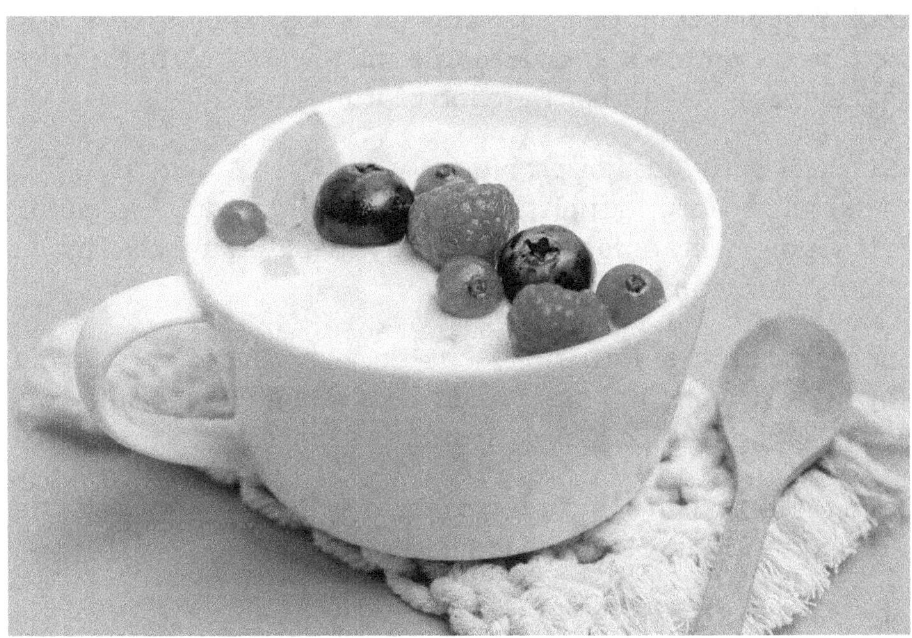

Fermented foods like yogurt, kimchi, sauerkraut, kefir and natto are rich in helpful bacteria called probiotics. These are the same bacteria that live in your gut and help your digestive system work properly.

Gut health and immunity are closely interrelated. Research has suggested that a healthy gut bacteria population can help your immune system tell the difference between healthy body cells and harmful invaders.

In one study, children who drank just 2.4 ounces (70 ml) of fermented milk daily had around 20% fewer childhood infectious diseases compared with the control group who didn't drink probiotics. If you don't regularly eat fermented foods, a probiotic supplement may be a good idea.

In another study of people infected with rhinovirus, those who took a supplement of the bacterium *Bifidobacterium animalis* had a stronger immune system response and lower levels of the virus in their nasal mucus than the control group did.

A typical daily dose of probiotics is between 1 and 10 billion CFUs (colony-forming units) daily. The key is to take these probiotic supplements or foods consistently to maintain a healthy gut and support your immune system.

It's best to eat probiotic-rich foods like yogurt or sauerkraut, but if you can't include those in your regular diet, you should consider supplements to improve your immune response .

Along with benefits include weight loss, digestive health, immune system, and other advantages.

This is an overview of the critical health benefits linked to probiotics.

<u>1. Probiotics aid in the balance of beneficial bacteria in the digestive system :</u>

Probiotics aid in the balance of friendly bacteria in the digestive system.Probiotics are beneficial bacteria that help the body function properly.These are live microorganisms that, when eaten, may provide health benefits.

The ability of probiotics to maintain the normal balance of gut bacteria is thought to be the source of these benefits. When there is an imbalance, there are too many harmful bacteria and not enough beneficial bacteria. It can occur as a result of disease, antibiotics, a bad diet, and other factors. Consequences can include stomach disorders, allergies, mental health issues, obesity, and other issues.

Fermented foods contain probiotics and are also used as supplements. Furthermore, the vast majority of people find them to be safe. and are also used as supplements. Furthermore, the vast majority of people find them to be safe.

2. Probiotics Can Help Prevent and Treat Diarrhea

Probiotics are well-known for their ability to avoid or lessen the severity of diarrhea. Antibiotics can cause diarrhea, which is a common side effect. Antibiotics can disrupt the balance of good and bad bacteria in the gut, causing this to happen. Probiotic use help to a lower risk of antibiotic-associated diarrhea in many studies.

Researchers discovered that taking probiotics decreased antibiotic-associated diarrhea by 42 percent in one trial.

Certain strains of probiotics will minimize the period of infectious diarrhea by an average of 25 hours, according to 35 studies.

Probiotics reduce the risk of travelers' diarrhea by 8%. They also reduced the risk of diarrhea from other causes in children by 57% and adults by 26%.

The effectiveness of probiotics varies depending on the form and dosage taken.

Lactobacillus rhamnosus, Lactobacillus casei, and the yeast Saccharomyces boulardii are the bacteria strains most frequently linked to a lower risk of diarrhea.

3. Supplementing with probiotics can help with a variety of mental health issues

A growing number of studies relate gut health to mental and emotional well-being.

Probiotic supplements help with a variety of mental health issues in both animal and human research.

According to a study, supplementing with Bifidobacterium and Lactobacillus strains for 1–2 months can boost anxiety, depression, autism, obsessive-compulsive disorder (OCD), and memory of 15 human studies.

For six weeks, one study followed 70 chemical staff. Many who ate 100 grams of probiotic yogurt or took a regular probiotic capsule saw improvements in their overall health, depression, anxiety, and stress.

In a survey of 40 depressed patients, there were also positive results.

4. Certain probiotic strains will help you maintain a healthy heart

By lowering LDL ("bad") cholesterol and blood pressure, probiotics can help keep your heart safe.

By breaking down bile in the gut, some lactic acid-producing bacteria can lower cholesterol.

Bile is a naturally occurring fluid that aids digestion and is primarily composed of cholesterol.

Probiotics can keep the bile from being reabsorbed in the gut, where it can reach the bloodstream as cholesterol, by breaking it down.

Probiotics can also help to reduce blood pressure.

Supplementation with more than eight weeks and 10 million colony-forming units (CFUs) per day helps to reduce blood pressure.

5. Probiotics can help to lessen the severity of allergies and eczema

Certain probiotic strains help children and babies with eczema.

In one study, children with probiotic-supplemented milk had more minor eczema symptoms than those given milk without probiotics.

Another research tracked the children of pregnant women who took probiotics. In the first two years of life, those children had an 83 percent lower chance of developing eczema.

However, there is still a poor correlation between probiotics and reduced eczema severity, and further research is required.

Some probiotics can also help people with milk or dairy allergies reduce their inflammatory responses.

6. Probiotics May Aid in the Reduction of Symptoms of Digestive Disorders

Inflammatory bowel disease affects over one million people in the United States.

In people with moderate ulcerative colitis, probiotics from the Bifidobacterium and Lactobacillus strains have improved symptoms.

Probiotics, on the other hand, tend not to affect Crohn's disease symptoms.

Probiotics, on the other hand, can be beneficial for other bowel disorders. Irritable bowel syndrome (IBS) symptoms can be alleviated, according to preliminary studies.

They've also cut the risk of severe necrotizing enterocolitis in half.

<u>7. Probiotics May Help Boost Your Immune System:</u>

Probiotics May Aid in Immune System Boosting Probiotics can aid in the strengthening of your immune system and inhibit the growth of harmful gut bacteria.

Additionally, some probiotics boost the body's natural antibody production. Immune cells such as IgA-producing cells, T lymphocytes, and natural killer cells may be grown as well.

Probiotics minimize the risk and length of respiratory infections. However, the testimony was of poor quality.

Another study of over 570 children discovered that taking Lactobacillus GG decreased the incidence and severity of respiratory infections by 17%.

<u>8. Probiotics help to loose weight:</u>

Probiotics May Aid in Immune System Boosting Probiotics can aid in the strengthening of your immune system and inhibit the growth of harmful gut bacteria.

Additionally, some probiotics boost the body's natural antibody production. Immune cells such as IgA-producing cells, T lymphocytes, and natural killer cells may be grown as well.

Probiotics minimize the risk and length of respiratory infections. However, the testimony was of poor quality.

Another study of over 570 children discovered that taking Lactobacillus GG decreased the incidence and severity of respiratory infections by 17%.

◆ ◆ ◆

7. REDUCE SUGAR INTAKE

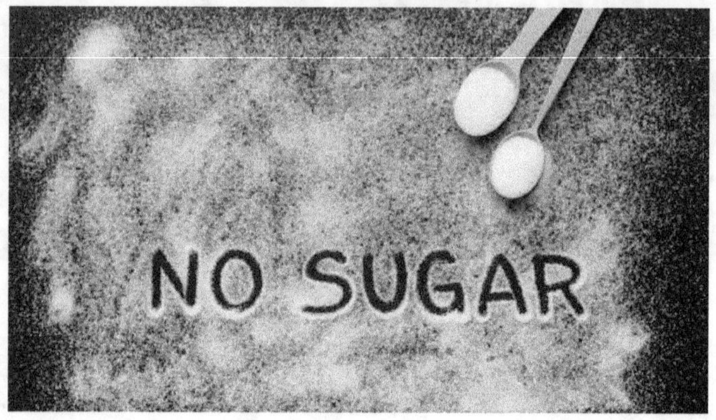

According to new studies, added sugars and refined foods can significantly lead to obesity, which can reduce the immune system's answer.

Obese people who had their annual flu shot were twice as likely as non-obese people to still get the flu afterward, according to a survey of about 1,000 people.

Inflammation can be reduced by reducing the sugar and refined food consumption.

It also helps you lose weight and lowers the risk of developing diseases like heart disease and type 2 diabetes.

Since all three diseases – obesity, diabetes, and heart disease – are known to wreak havoc on your immune system, try to keep your sugar consumption to 5% or less of your total daily caloric intake.

On a 2,000-calorie-per-day diet, you can consume no more than two tablespoonfuls (25 grammes) of sugar in a single day. Reducing your intake of sugar and refined foods will help you lose weight while also boosting your immune system.

What is the problem with added sugar?

Sugar is an essential carbohydrate that the body transforms into glucose and uses for energy in all of its types. However, the impact on your body and overall health is dependent on the kind of sugar you consume.

Added sugar offers no nutrients to your body, which is why it is sometimes referred to as 'empty calories,' which contribute to weight gain and obesity.

Too much sugar can cause various issues, ranging from difficulty concentrating, mood swings, rapid drops and rises in blood sugar, inflammation in the body, and chronic illnesses such as heart disease and diabetes.

According to the FDA, added sugar does not account for more than 10% of a person's daily calorie intake. However, the World Health Organization (WHO) decreased this figure from 10% to 5%. WHO recommends no more than five teaspoons of sugar for an adult with a regular BMI.

However, the guideline excludes naturally occurring sugar in fresh fruits, vegetables, milk, and whole grains, since these foods are considered to contain less sugar and have other health benefits. Added sugars, not naturally occurring sugar, are causing concern among physicians.

<u>Foods to Stay Away From If You're On A Sugar-Free Diet</u>

Pastries for breakfast (muffins, coffee cake)

Goods made from flour (cookies, cakes)

Sorbet and ice cream

Crackers and baked beans

Tacos (tacos)

Frozen rice entrees in a box

Cereals (bread, rice, and pasta)

Processed foods

Anything with sugar specified in the ingredients list or on the nutrition facts label

<u>Drinks To Avoid</u>

Soda

Fruit juices

Favored coffee, milk, tea

Hot chocolate

Tonic water

Cocktails

Liqueurs

Any other sugar-sweetened beverage

How To Survive A Sugar-Free Diet:

1. To begin, instead of sugar, add fresh or dried fruits to your cereal or oatmeal.

Fruits, with their sweet flavor and excellent taste, will make your breakfast even more delicious.

Nuts are another perfect way to make your oatmeal more appealing. Nutrients, calcium, and essential omega-3 fatty acids abound in hazelnuts, almonds, and cashews. Don't fall into the breakfast cereal pit when thinking about making breakfast on a no-sugar diet: most granolas and breakfast cereals sold as "good" are high in sugar. Cooking cereals by yourself is a much better bet.

2. Second, instead of sugar, use extracts such as almond, vanilla, lime, or lemon.

If fruits and fruit extracts aren't enough to satisfy your sweet tooth, some sweeteners might be able to help. Stevia, for example, has almost no calories and has a beneficial effect on blood sugar levels in people with diabetes. Erythritol and xylitol are less well-known but equally suitable alternatives.

These are low-calorie, natural sweeteners derived from fruits. In general, however, sweeteners can be used as a temporary rather than a permanent solution for your sugar-free diet.

3. If you're on a sugar-free diet and tired of plain water, tea, and sugar-free coffee, consider making lemon water. Lemon water is a straightforward and nutritious drink that will wake you up in the morning and get you ready for a great day.

Add Mint and cucumber to your bath. It's worth mentioning that substitute with fresh juices for unhealthy sodas.

If you're trying to cut down on sugar, this isn't the best choice. Although juices are rich in vitamins, they are also high in sugar and, unlike fresh fruits, do not give you a feeling of fullness.

4. Mindfull eating : Sugar cravings can be intense, and changing one's eating habits is often necessary. Mindful eating is a subset of mindfulness meditation that involves various activities to improve your relationship with food and allow you to savor each bite slowly and deliberately.

The key aim of mindful eating is to regain control over your eating habits by avoiding emotional overeating and boredom eating.

As a result, mindful eating will help you lose weight and encourage your attempts to adhere to a sugar-free diet.

5. Finally, instead of sugar, use spices such as ginger or cinnamon.

8. STRESS

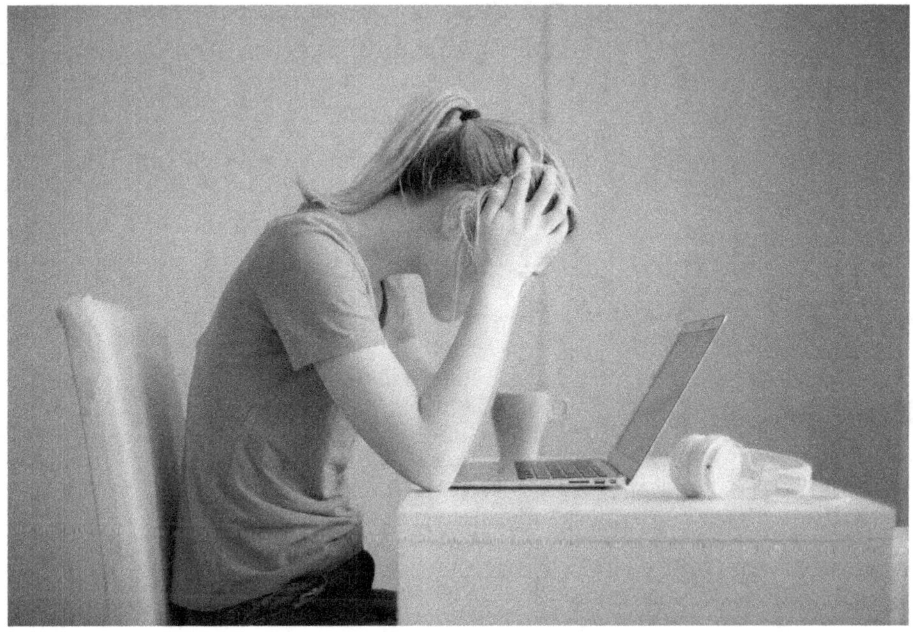

Your immune system and your mental health are inextricably linked.

Anxiety and stress are lousy germ fighters. According to studies, having anxious thoughts for as little as half an hour will lower your immune responseStress makes it much more difficult to battle viruses and bacteria. When you're stressed, your body produces cytokines, which are molecules that cause inflammation and can lower your immune response.

When you have chronic stress or anxiety, the body produces

stress hormones that weaken the immune system.

According to research, if you're nervous, you're more likely to catch a cold. Healthy adults exposed to the cold virus in one sample were then quarantined and tracked for five days.

Stressed people were twice as likely to become ill. "People who are depressed are often less likely to pay attention to behaviors, such as eating well and having enough sleep, which can impair immunity.

There's also evidence that long-term sadness weakens the immune system.

This effect will last up to six months, and it can last much longer if the grief is severe or long-lasting.

You can't stop tension or sadness, but you can use techniques to help handle it.

According to a report, adults who had a regular workout regimen or practiced mindfulness therapy were less likely to get sick with a respiratory infection – or, if they did, missed fewer days at work.

Long-term sadness weakens the immune system.

This effect will last for up to six months, and it can last even longer if the grief is extreme or prolonged.

You can't avoid tension or depression, but you can manage it with strategies.

Adults who exercised regularly or practiced mindfulness therapy were less likely to get sick with a respiratory infection – or, if they did, missed fewer days at work, according to a study.

The immune system's ability to combat antigens reduces when

nervous. As a result, we are more vulnerable to infections.

The stress hormone corticosteroid reduces the immune system's effectiveness (e.g., lowers the number of lymphocytes).

Stress may also indirectly impact the immune system because people can use unhealthy coping mechanisms to relieve stress, such as alcohol and smoking.

Headaches, respiratory illness (e.g., the flu), cardiovascular disease, diabetes, asthma, and gastric ulcers are related to stress.

What does a person's stress response entail?
When you are exposed to a stressor, a series of events arise before you even know you are in a stressful situation.
It's a complicated chain of events that causes the body to release a flood of hormones that cause physiological changes, such as:

1.Your heart rate and blood pressure rise, preparing you to fight by pushing blood to your muscles, heart, and other organs (or flee).

2. To give you more control, blood sugar, and fat from temporary storage sites.

3. You begin to breathe more quickly and inhale more oxygen. The additional oxygen boosts your alertness and sharpens your senses.

4. Your pupils dilate, allowing you to take in more light and see better.

5. The pain is dulled, allowing you to focus on what you need to do.

6. The body redistributes resources so that you can focus more

energy on survival processes and less on digestion, tissue repair, and immune functions.

<u>Stress management in real-time:</u>

1.Your body needs you to be able to react if anything stressful occurs. Here are some things you can do right now to assist the body in completing the stress cycle.

2.Take a stroll through the neighborhood.

3.Physical activity may assist in the management of excess energy.

4. Take a walk outside. Nature helps you change your perspective and relax.

5. Consult with family and friends. Talking about the situation will offer emotional comfort and a fresh outlook, making it less stressful.

6. Laugh regularly. Find something else to joke about if you can't laugh at your situation. Laughter will make you happier and help your brain function better.

◆ ◆ ◆

9. NO SMOKING

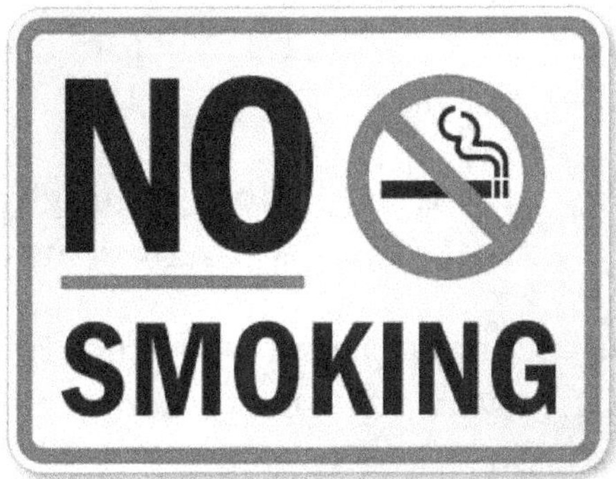

Smoking harms your lungs, which are two of your body's key entry points. nicotine reduces the capacity of your lungs to combat infection and increase inflammation.

"chemicals emitted by cigarette smoke – carbon monoxide, nicotine, nitrogen oxides, and cadmium – can interfere with the growth and function of immune cells, including T-cells, cytokines, and B-cells."

Infections are exacerbated by smoking, especially in the lungs (like pneumonia, flu, and tuberculosis).

And even a single night of binge drinking will impair your body's ability to combat germs for up to 24 hours. Drinking too much will harm the body's ability to repair damage over time.

Alcoholics are more susceptible to liver disease, influenza, tuberculosis, and some cancers. Stick to one drink a day for women and two drinks a day for men if you're going to indulge with caution.

Tobacco use and excessive alcohol use are also unhealthy in several respects.

Your immune system is one of the things you might not have noticed.

There are many methods for quitting smoking and drinking. If you're having trouble, see your doctor for professional advice about how to get better again.

According to Study, even a single bout of binge drinking will reduce the immune system's response to invading pathogens.

Study states that alcohol's primary metabolite, acetaldehyde, impairs ciliary activity in the lungs, rendering them more susceptible to bacterial and viral invasion.

According to study, alcohol impairs the mechanism of targeting and breaking down bacteria and viruses, making people who abuse alcohol more susceptible to infection.

10. SUPPLEMENTS

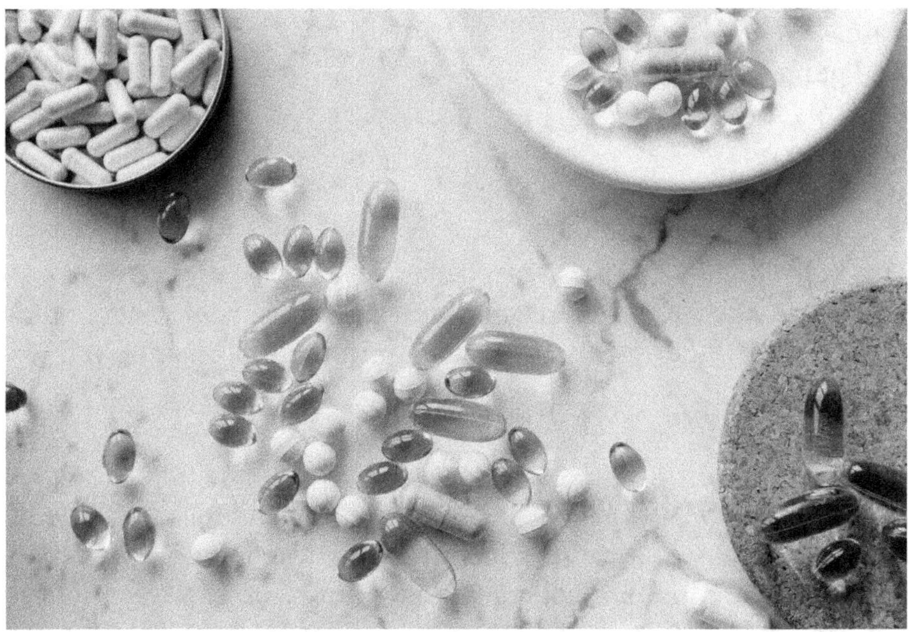

According to a dietitian ,"a fully stable immune system relies on a consistent healthy diet over time." "It's like getting ready for a fight and preparing the body so it can throw a strong punch when viruses, bacteria, and toxins strike. Other lifestyle habits, such as daily exercise and adequate sleep, will help you prepare for the fight." With a few exceptions, it's preferable to get vitamins and minerals from food rather than pills.

Dietician offers some advice on how to get some of the most important vitamins and minerals for a healthy immune system:

1. Vitamin C:

Vitamin C can help to prevent or shorten the duration of infections. Citrus fruits are one of the best sources, but did you know there are others? Yes, that is right! Dietician suggests that you do the following:

Spinach.
Kale.
Bell peppers.
Brussels sprouts.
Strawberries.
Papaya.

Fun fact: Since vitamin C can be found in so many foods, most people do not need to take supplements unless their doctor recommends it. Before taking any vitamin C supplements, talk to your doctor.

2. Vitamin E:

Vitamin E, like vitamin C, is a potent antioxidant that aids in the fight against infection. This vital vitamin, which is involved in nearly 200 biochemical reactions in your body, is essential for the proper functioning of your immune system. Consider high-fat plant foods to get your vitamin E, such as:
Almonds.
Peanuts/peanut butter.
Sunflower seeds.
Oils such as sunflower, safflower, and soybean oil.
Hazelnuts.

3. Vitamin A:

Vitamin A is an infection-fighting vitamin that can be found in two forms: preformed in animal foods like fish, meat, and dairy, and plant carotenoids. Preformed vitamin A is abundant in tuna.

When it comes to carotenoids, go for the bright colours:

Carrots.
Sweet potatoes.
Pumpkin.
Butternut squash.
Cantaloupe.
Dark green leafy vegetables.

4. Vitamin D:

It's also known as the sunshine vitamin, and it's one of the most essential and effective nutrients for immune system support. There are a few food options, but they include:

Salmon.
Mackerel.
Tuna.
Sardines.
Milk, orange juice, and cereals are all fortified with vitamin D. In general, we get many of your vitamins from food, but vitamin D may be an exception. Consult your doctor to see if you need a supplement.

5. Folate/folic acid:

Folate is the natural form, while folic acid is the synthetic form, often added to foods for their health benefits. Add more beans and lentils to your diet daily, as well as leafy green vegetables, to get more folate. Another delectable source is avocado. Folic acid is in fortified foods (check the label first).

Enriched pasta.
Enriched bread.
Enriched rice.

6. Iron:

Many immune system processes depend on iron, which helps your body bring oxygen to cells. It is available in a variety of shapes and sizes. Heme iron (also known as iron from animal products) absorbed by the body and in abundance in the following foods:

Red meat (limit to smaller amounts and less often).
Chicken.
Turkey.
Canned sardines.
Oysters.
Clams.
Mussels.
Canned light tuna.
If you're a vegetarian, have no fear. You can still find iron in:

Beans.
Broccoli.
Kale.
Iron-fortified cereals.

7. Selenium:

Selenium appears to have a significant impact on the immune system, making it essential for infection prevention. Except for Brazil nuts, which provide more than 100% of the daily value in just one nut, animal foods are the best sources. However, too much of something can be harmful, so limit yourself to one to two of these a day. Look for selenium in the following foods:

Seafood (tuna, halibut, sardines).
Meat and liver.
Poultry.
Cottage cheese.

8. Zinc:

Zinc is for the development of new immune cells. It's primarily found in animal foods but can also find it in some vegetarian foods:

Oysters.
Crab.
Lean meats and poultry.
Baked beans.
Yogurt.
Chickpeas.

If you can't get fresh food, go for frozen.

You can not always obtain high-quality fresh produce depending on where you live and the time of year.

Remember that buying frozen food is a good choice and can be very convenient in our time-crunched world. And frozen food will help the immune system.

"Frozen fruits and vegetables are frozen at 'peak' ripeness, which ensures they have the same nutritional value as their fresh counterparts, "Rather than frozen foods with added sugars or sodium, prefer pure frozen foods."

All of these vitamins and supplements will boost the immune system. If you're thinking about taking vitamins or other supplements in pill form, talk to your doctor first.

CONCLUSION

The immune system is a wonderful part of the human body.

It identifies and combats germs such as viruses, bacteria, and fungi.

It also fights disease-causing changes in the body by neutralising toxic compounds.

For Everyday Health, study says, "Think of the immune system as an ensemble." "You want every instrument and every player in the orchestra to work at their best for the best performance." You don't need one musician to start playing at double speed or one instrument to start playing at maximum volume.

Your immune system is in the same boat. There are a variety of things you can do to strengthen your immune system and aid your body in the battle against disease.

Exercise regularly, quit smoking and drinking, get enough sleep, and control your stress are all things you've heard your whole life.

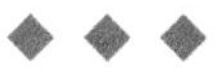

RESOURCES

Here are links that it will help you:

https://www.healthline.com/nutrition/immune-boosting-supplements

https://www.webmd.com/cold-and-flu/ss/slideshow-how-you-suppress-immune-system

https://www.health.harvard.edu/staying-healthy/how-to-boost-your-immune-system

https://www.healthgrades.com/right-care/coronavirus/10-tips-to-boost-your-immunity-during-covid-19

https://pharmeasy.in/blog/9-immunity-boosting-herbs-to-beat-covid-19/

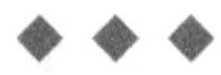